The Sarcastic Girl's Guide to Pregnancy

Or

Oh, You Thought This Was Going to Be Fun?

Sarah Obloy

ISBN:1979968152
ISBN-13:9781979968157

DEDICATION

To Little Chainsaw – without whom I would have had no reason to write this book and for Patrick, without whom I wouldn't have had Chainsaw.

CONTENTS

Author's Note

I started this as a blog when I got pregnant, as a way to vent - since I was pretty sure that my friends were all really sick of me complaining all the time. I'm the child of a Child Development/Parenting teacher, so I figured I was ready for pregnancy. I know all the stages, I've read all the books, and I lived through my mom being pregnant with my three brothers. "I've got this," I thought to myself.

Boy, was I wrong.

The book *What to Expect When You're Expecting* leaves a lot out. A LOT. A ridiculous amount, even. I was 100% not prepared for the parasitic invasion that was my firstborn. Every pregnancy is different, and I'm sure there are some magical unicorn moms out there that had textbook, perfect pregnancies. I'm not one of those moms. So here are my thoughts and experiences, in hopes that if you, like me, are not ready for all this, you can get some insight into all the madness that is pregnancy and tiny humans. And if you're not crazy enough to join me on the preggo train, maybe it'll be good for a laugh.

Sarah

October 2017

1
SO, YOU GOT YOURSELF KNOCKED UP

So, you're pregnant. Knocked up. With child. Infected by a growing parasite. Any other hip and with it slang terms for the miracle of growing new life.

Now what?

If you live near, or are always around, single people or couples who like you have dogs instead of kids, chances are the majority of your pregnancy knowledge comes from TV, movies, listening to your family talk about how much your mom went through having you, and the incredible madness that is the show "I Didn't Know I was Pregnant". This show, by the way, once you've been pregnant for a while, becomes completely unbelievable. I find myself yelling at the TV "seriously Judy*? You thought that the constant nausea, mood swings, tight fitting pants and bras, and that weird kicking in your stomach were just normal "female troubles"? Not to mention that pesky lack of a period?" I know I've had some gnarly PMS, but being pregnant is a whole different ballgame - mostly because my uterus and body hated me for a totally different reason.

Side note: those pesky uteruses - they're angry at you when you don't let your egg implant itself in it, and they're angry at you when you do. They're just never freaking happy.

For everyone I know, being more than a few days late, or feeling funky (that's a clinical term, by the way) or being super tired merits running out to the store and buying a stick to pee on. Not an actual stick, of course, but one of those ridiculously priced pink boxes in the "lady" section of the drugstore. My brother says you can also pee on a rabbit or something, and if it dies, that means you're pregnant. But I think he was just trying to get me to traumatize an innocent bunny. But I digress. Then, if you haven't been trying to have a kid, there is the usual sigh of relief when that second line does appear. If you have been trying, your reaction is going to be different.

But now you find yourself in possession of a positive test. This might be an accident, or a surprise, or you may have been trying for said result. Now what? My previous pregnancy experience (TV and movies) taught me to expect dewy skin and a general pregnancy glow that others could spot, an adorable round baby bump, the need to pee a lot, cute little baby kicks, and some early morning vomiting. Turns out I was right about the peeing…and that's about it. They did not prepare me from the 9 months that were to follow - not at all.

Looking back, I ask myself if anything could have prepared me for what lay ahead. Honestly, I think that if someone had told me what was going to happen, 1) I probably would have laughed and told them it couldn't possibly be that bad, and 2) thought long and hard about deciding that having a tiny human. Thankfully, I didn't know, because otherwise I might have lost out on my tiny terror.

*Name made up, because all the names on those shows are made up anyway.

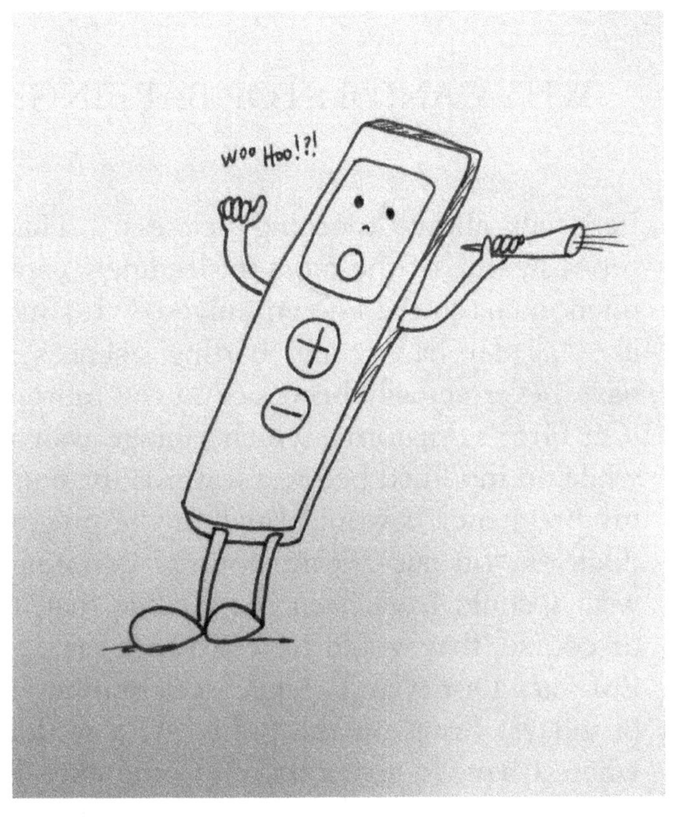
Woo Hoo!?!

2
WHY CAN'T I STOP BARFING?

Let's talk about "morning sickness". This is seriously one of the most misleadingly named phenomena in the known universe. It's more like "all day nausea and barfing sickness". I have never actually been sick in the morning. On Grey's Anatomy, which I binge watched while on modified bed rest towards the end of my pregnancy, I would laugh at the pregnant doctor's "on cue" 9 am bout of vomiting. I wish I could have been regular like that, but of course, that would have made it easy. 11 PM at Disneyland while celebrating my birthday? Bring on the puke. At a wedding where I have to give a toast? Vomit city. But when I'm in the comfort of my own home, with easy access to my toothpaste and toothbrush? No way. It's ridiculous.

I have heard tales of these magical women that sailed through their nine months of hosting an alien with no problems. They ate what they wanted, went where they wanted, and didn't fear spontaneous barf at work. Most of us aren't that lucky. My cupboard at work is stocked with anti-nausea suckers, prescription no-barf pills, tummy calming tea, and bubbly water...along with toothpaste, a toothbrush, and peppermints (because mouthwash would make me throw up again. Besides the aforementioned wedding disaster, where I RAN out the door the minute I finished my speech to worship the porcelain god (does anyone even use that term anymore? It's super 90's), I have had to frantically find people to watch my classroom full of children while I hurried to the restroom. One time I couldn't find anyone so I had to throw up in the trash can right in front of my room, since schools tend to frown on both leaving children unattended and throwing up in front of them. It's a catch 22.

Doesn't being pregnant sound awesome? It's the most fun – especially when you spend you holidays in party cities like Las Vegas because almost your whole family decided to live there. Obviously, giant alcoholic slushy drinks and fancy cocktails with blooming flowers are out. This isn't the 1960's, and they frown on expectant mothers boozing it up and smoking in bars. So what else is there to do in Vegas? Well, there are always slot machines, I thought. Except, of course, the smell of the casino I met my friends in was so pungent – an odious mix of artificial flower spray, cigarette smoke, and desperation – that I got super nauseous and was afraid to stand back up after I sat down at a machine because I was worried that I would become Mr. Creosote. (Side note: If you don't get the Creosote reference, or have never seen Meaning of Life, stop what you're doing RIGHT NOW and go watch it. Seriously. I'll wait.)

According to every pregnancy guide I've read (and I've read many), this horrible nausea is supposed to disappear as you enter the second trimester, also known as "the period where people can finally tell that you're pregnant". To them I say "Pshaw!" I don't know about that. At the time of this writing, I am one day from that magical trimester mark…and I've had to resist throwing up twice today. I'm supposed to magically wake up tomorrow with a perfect constitution? I'll blame you, pregnancy books, when I dig into those delicious nachos tomorrow at lunch and then turn into a barf machine during my one o'clock class.

PS. I totally blamed the books. I threw up for nine months straight. I never got to eat those nachos.

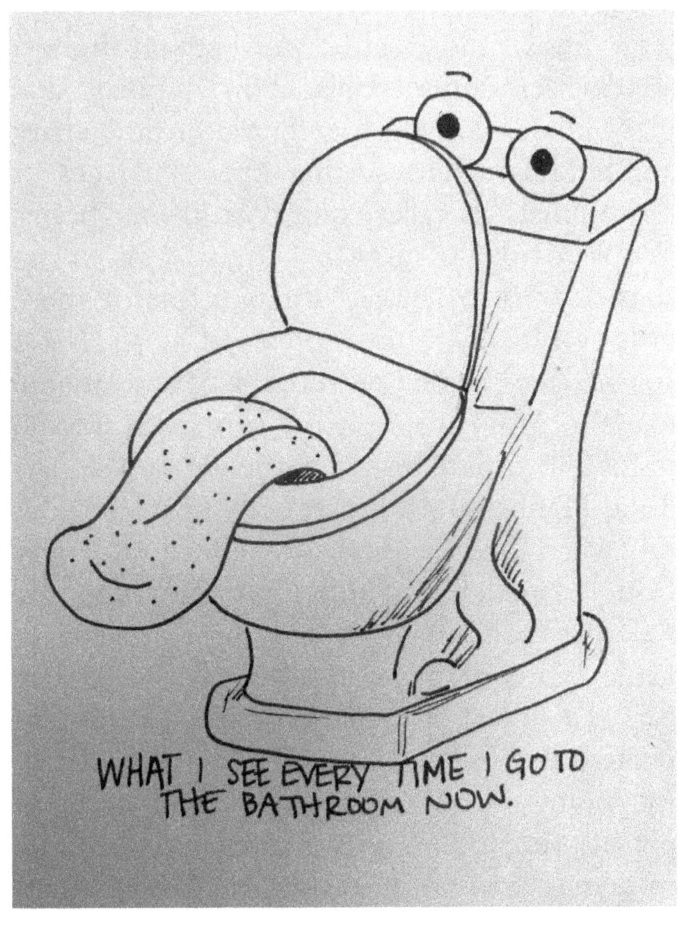

WHAT I SEE EVERY TIME I GO TO
THE BATHROOM NOW.

3
WHORE MOANS…OR, WHY CAN'T I STOP FUCKING CRYING?

You know those girls who cry at things? Budweiser commercials about puppies and giant horses coming together after time apart, Sarah McLaughlin singing over the faces of sad animals in cages, tiny pigs in rain boots, people dying in movies – those girls cry at these and many more. I'm not one of those girls. (Actually, I am not a girl at all, but a full-fledged woman with the debt and student loans to prove it.) I shed a tear when Kermit is forced to part from his friends in Muppets Take Manhattan, but that's about it. I didn't cry when Dobby died at the end of Harry Potter (spoiler for those of you who are woefully behind), or when Beth croaked in Little Women (she was boring anyway). I've NEVER cried at a commercial. I cry for relative deaths, and when I am frustrated to the point of no return and my choices are physical exploding into a million tiny pieces, or crying. I'm not into weeping. Happy tears do not escape my dry, emotionless eyes. Please note that I'm not disparaging those girls in ANY way. Many of my friends are those girls. Crying is healthy and should never be judged. I'm just not a crier - or a hugger, but that's a whole different story.

And the, it happened - the hormones. I've heard the stories, and seen the movies where the pregnant lady bursts into tears because she spilled her iced tea, saw a picture of a cute baby, or some other stupid, trivial event.

"That won't be me," I thought. "I have a heart of stone, and no tears shall pass!" (I said that last bit in my best Gandalf voice.) Basically, I jinxed myself, because the hormone gods heard my overconfident statements and cursed me. I realized I was screwed when I was watching one of my favorite ridiculous crime shows — you know, the one with the ginger guy who likes dramatic pauses and taking off his sunglasses to emphasize his point — and someone got shot and killed; now, in my hormonal defense, it was a main character, not just the corpse of the day. I found myself sobbing, lying in my bed clutching a handful of Kleenex as the water leaked from my eyes. My husband popped his head into the room and asked me if I was crying. "No!" I insisted. It was totally allergies. Until the next day, when I spilled my drink and burst into tears. And then teared up at a commercial full of sad children. Holy shit. I've become that girl.

It's getting worse as the alien spawn grows inside me – just to warn you. A flashback post on Facebook turned me into a sobbing ball of sadness, because it was Christmas and we didn't have that house anymore. I get sad when I watch TV. My pants wouldn't button up anymore and the tears came. I turned off a show because a little kid got kidnapped. A freaking Disney movie made me cry.

Now, I know I'm a big sobbing ball of hormones, but I try to ignore it. Case in point. Alan Rickman, one of my all-time favorite actors, just died, so I'm sad. Normally, I would not cry at an actor's death - I'd just be depressed and draw some fan art. Now, I know that random things make me cry, and yet I still decide that it would be a great idea to a) watch the last Harry Potter movie where Snape dies. (Spoiler, but seriously- the book's been out for a million years.) I also decide to start listening to the audiobook versions of the books. As a result, not only did I spend almost 2 hours after the movie crying on my pillow about Snape, I also showed up to work red eyed and teary for weeks on end….because I listen to books on my commute to work, and towards the end of the Potter series J.K. Rowling turns into freaking George R. R. Martin. It's freaking ridiculous. I can watch the most gory horror movie without batting an eye, but a cartoon elephant-cotton candy-thing fades out of existence and I'm a wreck. Hormones are for the birds.

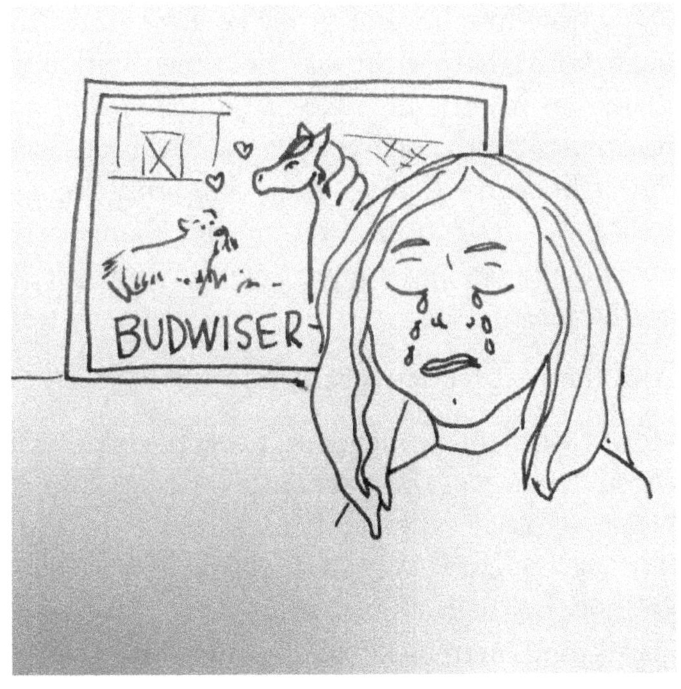

4
FAT PANTS –
A GIRL'S BEST FRIEND

I'm not a skinny girl. My body role model is Mindy Kaling. If I could look like Mindy, my life would be sweet. My regular jeans are someone else's fat pants - you know, the ones where they put both legs in one leg hole to show how much weight they've lost? And I'm okay with that, most of the time – mostly thanks to my friends who are super into body positivity and positive mental attitudes. I didn't like myself for a long time, but thanks to lots of reflection, attempts to change my inner dialogue, and support from my people, I got better.

And then…pregnancy struck.

Here's one thing they don't teach you in all those "what to expect when you're expecting" books – Bloat. It's like being on your period, but way worse. Within the first ten weeks, your poor belly (no matter what size you started out) starts to expand – but not because of your alien invader. He's only an inch or so long at most. No, it's the dreaded bloat. All those girls who post their "baby bump" at 10 week - just stop it. That's like posting a picture of you right at the beginning of your period. Arching your back doesn't turn that bloat into a baby…time does that. I didn't look pregnant until I was at about 36 weeks, but my clothes stopped fitting almost instantly. Thanks a lot, bloat!

Which brings us to fat pants. I knew I was in bloaty baby trouble when I was about 6 weeks along and had to go out of state for a work conference. Not thinking "hey, my 2 millimeter long baby is totally going to be affecting me right now" (and having not been warned this was going to happen) I packed my outfits like I would for any other conference during fall – jeans, t-shirt, sneakers. Imagine my surprise when, on that first morning in the hotel, I pulled on my jeans – and they didn't button. Like not even close - there was a good 2 inches of gap between the button and the hole. The hotel and surrounding areas (and especially the police) frown upon ladies wandering their halls and streets with no pants on, and I really didn't want to spend my time in a Dallas jail. I spent precious time wracking my brain – could I turn my bed sheet into a toga, or perhaps a fashionable skirt? No, my underwear were bright pink, and the sheet was white. That was a recipe for disaster. The hotel gift shop only sold extremely overpriced bedazzled dresses and sweatshirts, and none of them came in plus size. Finally, I spotted my salvation: a rubber band. I quickly looped that shit through my buttonhole and connected it the button. Voila! Instant fat pants. Thank goodness I always wear a tank top under my shirt - I was able to hide my MacGyver skills and go out in public. That trip, I discovered how hard it is to get emergency clothes in the middle of a downtown area when you don't have a car. It's not an experience I want to ever have to repeat.

As soon as I returned home, I tried to find other, more permanent solutions to my fat pants problem. "I'm not even 3 months pregnant", I thought, "There is no way I should be buying maternity clothes." I decided to invest in a belly band, so I could go to work without buttoning up my pants. It seemed like a good idea, but I have hips for days and a big butt, so it just kept rolling up, exposing my unbuttoned pants to the world. Then I discovered a magical button extender that came with a handy dandy extra piece of fabric, so that even if my shirt rode up, no one would be able to see my panties.

More importantly, I embraced yoga pants. When you are all preggo bloaty (or later, when your bloat has turned into baby), yoga pants are the shit. They are stretchy, comfortable and don't have those annoying buttons and zippers that dig into your expanding belly. Their waistbands are fabric, and can be rolled up to cover your pooch or pushed down below it – either is magical. Plus, unlike the Lula Roe leggings I broke down and bought later, they won't break the bank….unless you shop at Lulu Lemon. (Also, what's with stores that start with "lu" being so freaking expensive?)

Fat pants make life more tolerable.

Now, wearing fat pants doesn't mean you ARE fat…every girl has those clothes that she breaks out when shark week hits. When you're pregnant, your whole closet becomes those clothes. Yoga pants. That oversized men's button up shirt you bought for western wear day at work. Roll waist maxi skirts. These are your friends.

Pack those super tight tops, form fitting dresses with zippers down the back, no-stretch skirts, and anything that isn't made of a soft jersey material away. Embrace the fat pants. Life is way more comfortable here.

Besides your belly, other things swell too…like your boobs. Literature says the average woman goes up a cup size while pregnant. This is awesome when you're a B cup, sure – but what if your boobs are already way larger than you'd like them? As it is, I can't buy half the bra styles at Victoria's Secret – because Victoria's secret is that she has tiny little perky boobs. I really don't want to have to turn to the depths of the internet in my search for gigantic bras. But, sure enough, those suckers swelled. I'm holding out, however. I'm going to keep shoving my honeydews into a cantaloupe sized bra until it's obscene, and they threaten to pop out in public. Because that's how I roll.

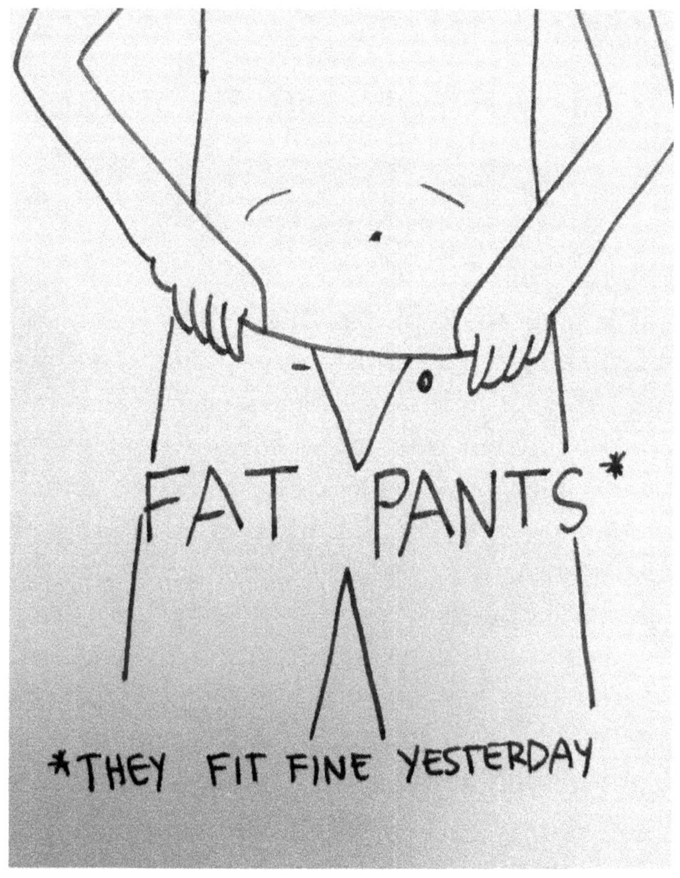

FAT PANTS*
*THEY FIT FINE YESTERDAY

5

ALL DOCTORS ARE VAMPIRES

Giving blood sucks. Sure, when you participate in a blood drive, they give you juice and cookies, and occasionally a t-shirt, but the appeal of that wears off after college…when you can afford to buy your own juice and cookies without letting someone stick needles into you like they're giant human leeches. I hate going to the doctor because they always want to stick needles into you. And I have really tiny, hard to find veins that like to roll, hide, collapse, or generally do whatever else they can to keep from getting stabbed with pointy things; I'm inevitably poked upwards of 4 times before anyone gets a successful blood draw any time I go to the doctor. In fact, the ONLY reason I like going to the dentist is because he doesn't try to take blood. After a visit to my doctor I always end up looking like an abused pincushion. Imagine my delight…..no, delight is the wrong word. Horror? That's more like it. Imagine my horror when I discovered that, as a pregnant lady, the doctors get to suck out my blood whenever they want. And by "whenever they want", I mean "all the time".

During my first visit to my friendly doctor man, he informed me that they would have to draw blood occasionally. I imagined a quick vial or two, and was completely fine with that. Imagine my surprise when I wandered down to the lab, and the nice technician pulls out 12 empty vials…all ready to be filled with my sweet precious blood. "Your veins are going to be plumper while you're pregnant, so it will be easier to draw blood," she lied to me with a straight face. I let her warm grandmotherly looks affect my judgment – after all, grandma wouldn't lie to me – and believed her as I stuck out my arm. Three technicians and 6 bruises later, they finally got their pint of blood. Add "plump veins" to the list of things people have lied about.

Since that initial visit, the doctor has found a way to separate me from my blood every time I go in. They need to check my liver. They need to check my flobberworms. They need to check my midichlorian levels. A different reason every time, but all of them an excuse to poke me with sharp things and steal my blood. By the end, I'll be like one of those pallid, on the brink of death waifs that Dracula left in his wake.

I'm convinced that they don't really need all that blood. My theory? The phlebotomists are really vampires, and pregnant lady blood is like a really nice zinfandel. They could drink that Two Buck Chuck from Trader Joes, but they'd much rather kick back with a delicious pint of my sweet, sweet preggo nectar. They stock their mini fridges with it. They use it as a base in their boeuf bourguignon. They bring out vials of lots of us to do tastings at their dinner parties. It's a secret world we know nothing about.

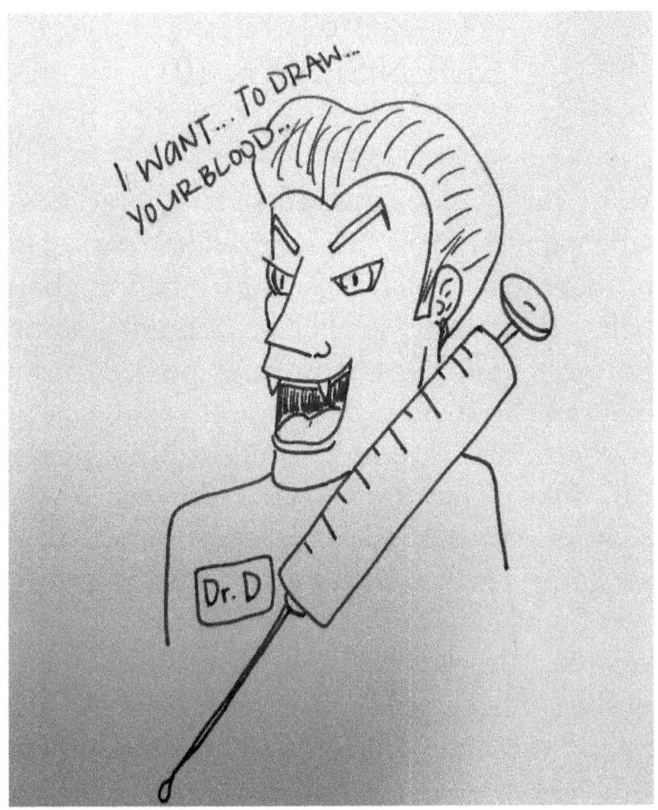

Actual image of my Doctor….at least what he looked like when he was stabbing me with needles.

6
ALIEN SPAWN 101

All of the books, apps, and various pieces of baby paraphernalia have provided expectant mothers with a plethora of information about their gestating spawn. Mothers across Pinterest and Instagram have posted proud pictures about how their bump is the size of an onion, or a pea, or a kumquat. But let's be real, folks. That tiny parasite growing in your belly is not an adorable strawberry, or a delicious peach. The reality is much weirder.

At the beginning, your baby resembles nothing even vaguely baby-looking. Usually, around the time you find out that you're with child, said child resembles a half chewed gummy bear, or perhaps a really gnarly tadpole, without the tail. (Unless your kid has a tail. Some do. We don't judge.) It's a tiny blob, albeit one that makes you super tired, super nauseous, and bloated. It's sucking all of your energy, your vital life force, so that it can transform itself from gummy bear mode to something that looks vaguely more humanoid. Because it is a parasite, folks. It gestates in your belly like the product of a face hugger (although its exit is decidedly less messy), draining your energy and blood flow so that it can grow. The only difference between your tiny human and the goo-dripping alien from Aliens is that your tiny person is a lot cuter and (hopefully) won't try to kill you. Oh, and way fewer teeth.

By three months, it has started to resemble a person more, especially in your ultrasound. In reality, it's a giant headed squishy with translucent skin and creepy eyelids. By the time it's fully developed, it's peeing and drinking the same fluids. If there was a person walking around that looked like your baby bean, you would run screaming down the street, not post pictures to Instagram and Facebook comparing it to blueberry.
Also, they steal your bones. This is a fact. Like a Tooth Fairy for your whole body, your alien spawn leeches your nutrients (which is why you need the dreaded pre-natal vitamins, and lots of calcium). If you don't get enough calcium, the baby will suck it out of you, like a diner at a fine restaurant sucks the marrow from the bones in his Osso Buco. And when I say 'from you' I mean your skeleton and teeth. If you're not on top of your vitamin game you could end up like the poor

townsfolk in The Tommyknockers. (For those of you who aren't big readers, The Tommyknockers is one of the lesser known works of Stephen King. It was made into a miniseries with Jimmy Smits and Marg Helgenberger, and its images of people's' teeth falling out haunts me to this day. If you haven't seen The Tommyknockers, you're missing out. It's awesome. And it will add to your distrust of dolls. If you can't find it on video, read the book. Reading is fundamental.)

Eventually, your tiny alien will start to resemble a cute squishy baby, at which time it's fully baked and can come out. Of course, what you can't tell from that 4D ultrasound you paid extra for is that your adorable bundle of joy is covered with fuzz. That's right, your sweet baby is a tiny Chewbacca. Thankfully, it all falls off before it's born, but still. It's a tiny fuzzling. After the birth, of course, there can be shockers. Your precious chicken nugget of a baby could have a super hairy butt (or shoulders, like mine did), a face full of pimples, or look like Winston Churchill. I'm not talking serious birth defects - those are no laughing matter. But a baby that emerges looking like Mr. Potato Head? I'm going to laugh. Sorry.

Aren't babies fun?

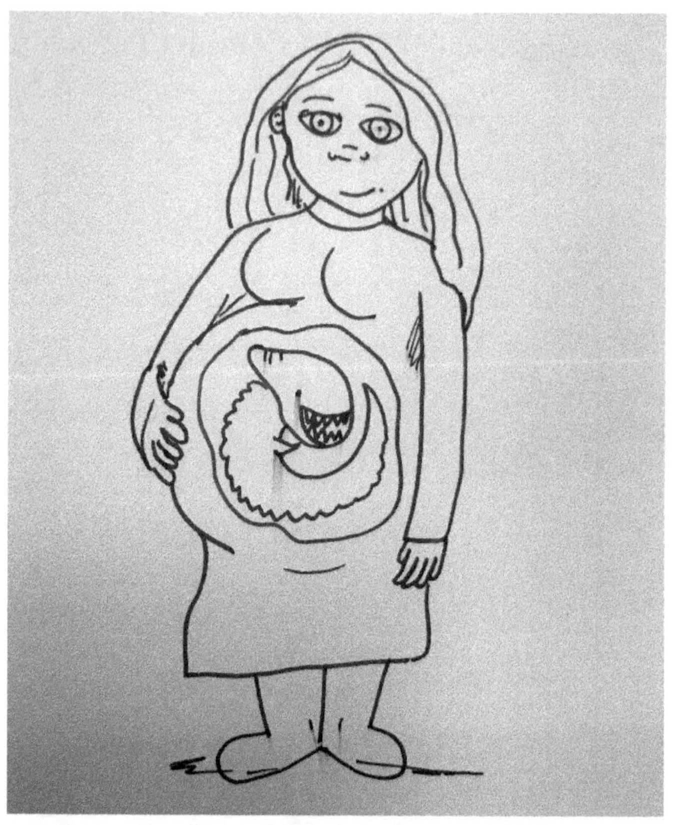

A Rough approximation of what's inside your belly.
I once posted on Facebook "7 weeks until the parasite emerges"....and got so much hate from someone in the comments. Whatever. She's my parasite, and I love her.

7
WHERE'S THE BEEF?

Let's talk about food for a minute. All the lovely pregnancy guides talk about how your nausea and sickness will pass after the 1st three months - it's like the second trimester is this golden period, where all of the sick and tired of that first 12 weeks is wiped away like your sins at a baptism. It sounds so lovely, doesn't it? I dreamt of that second trimester as I was huddled over the toilet at work or on the sofa, clutching my pillow, actively trying not to vomit. "I will be one of those happy pregnant ladies yet!" I kept lying to myself.

When I hit 3 months, I was really excited. "Finally!" I thought. "I'll be able to eat all the foods again!" Little did I know that this was not to be the case. I headed into the Christmas break still unable to eat most things. The smell alone of most foods made me nauseous. While my family went out and celebrated, I spent Christmas Eve curled up on a bed (when not barfing) because I had dared to try a bite of sausage at a party earlier that night. For Christmas dinner I ate 3 bites of mashed potatoes and some bread. In my 4th month, when I should have been able to keep my pace during the Star Wars 10K, I was instead the last person to cross the finish line….because I had to stop and throw up in the middle of the race - not, as you may assume, because I was out of shape, but because I stopped at the water station and drank a 3 oz. cup full of water. The next day I volunteered to cheer on the half marathoners, and as I watched pregnant woman after pregnant woman run by me, I was so freaking jealous of their ability to run and their apparent lack of nausea problems. I couldn't even drink water without it making me want to throw up.

I read all these articles about "eating healthy for your baby" and see all these moms online working out and making these super gorgeous healthy meals for themselves, and here I am. My prenatal yoga DVD just sits, because I have zero energy when I get home for work. My diet consists of rice, beans, cheese, tater tots, pickles (in any form), some fruit, and green juice…because basically anything else I try makes me super nauseous or gives me cramps. And don't get me started on foods that smell. My poor beleaguered husband has to deal with cooking dinner….only to have me either reject it outright because it smells gross, or take one bite and push it away because it does not sit well with me (or just straight up tastes gross). My parasite has forced me to become a vegetarian. Last night, my best friend brought over donuts….and I couldn't kiss my man because I could taste and smell donut on his lips – and it tasted like dead things.

Food has been banned from my classroom as well, because I can smell the students Hot Cheetos, and it makes me want to hurl. A kid brought in corn nuts, and overwhelming stench of rotting corpses and feet made me dash outside and puke in a bush.

Here's hoping that this gets better at some point, because I would kill for a regular meal.

PS. It didn't.

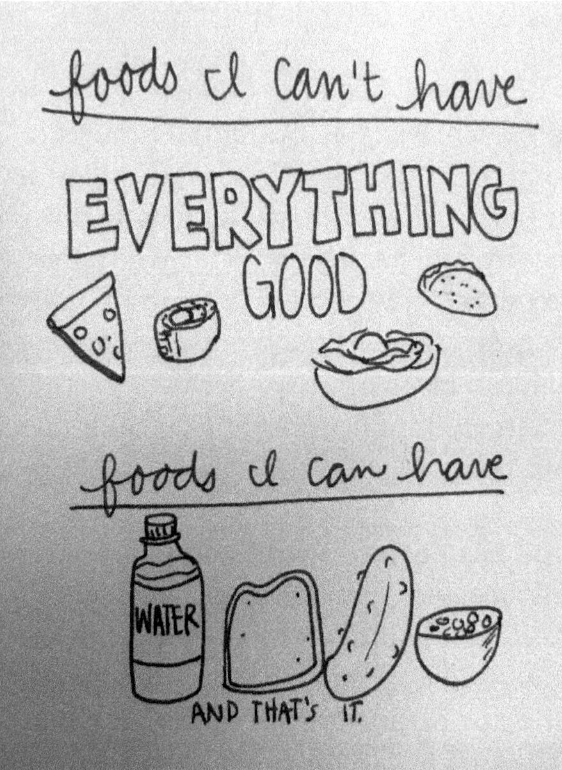

foods I can't have
EVERYTHING GOOD
foods I can have
WATER
AND THAT'S IT.

8
EVERYBODY POOPS…..EXCEPT YOU.

So, if the constant nausea (or, if you're one of the lucky ones, 3 months of nausea) and the barfing weren't enough to make you want to run out and join the pregnancy train, maybe a strong case of the "holy-shit-why-can't-I-poop"s will. That's right, your old friend constipation. Now, if you're a normal, healthy person who doesn't eat a lot of shit (not actual shit, mind you, because that would just be disgusting, but processed shit, like candy and white bread), perhaps constipation isn't something you've experienced before. But for the lucky pregnant lady, it becomes a way of life. Because everyone gets to poop – except you. I almost had that made into a t shirt - complete with a tiny Ghostbusters-style no poop emoji.

After I enjoyed several days of not being able to go, even if I used the magical unicorn poop-inducing machine that is the Squatty Potty, I found myself in the one section of the drugstore I had never before needed to peruse: the ex-lax and fiber aisle. Being in

this aisle made me feel about a hundred (mostly because I already feel about seventy, what with the lack of sleep and the exhaustion and the nausea, and the aisle added another 30 years). I found myself at the register not with my usual tube of mascara and 20 oz. diet Dr. Pepper, but with some Metamucil and fiber plus. That night, and for several days after, I very grudgingly mixed a scoop or 2 with orange juice, hoping that Mary Poppins was right and that a spoonful of sugar would really help the medicine go down. And once it did, and I was as regular as I could be, I stopped…and then learned to my horror that once I stopped taking this medicine, I was right back where I started. So now, instead of enjoying a late night cup of tea, I take my grainy, artificially orange flavored medicine, and continue to count the days until I can go back to being a normal person. We call it my "poop juice". My husband walked in as I'm drinking my gritty beverage. "Honey, what is that nasty stuff", he asked. "It's my poop juice!" I said cheerfully. "Want some?"
Spoiler: he didn't.
But now I can holler at him from wherever I am and ask him to make me some poop juice….and isn't that what being married is all about?

Or, You Thought This Was Going To Be Easy?

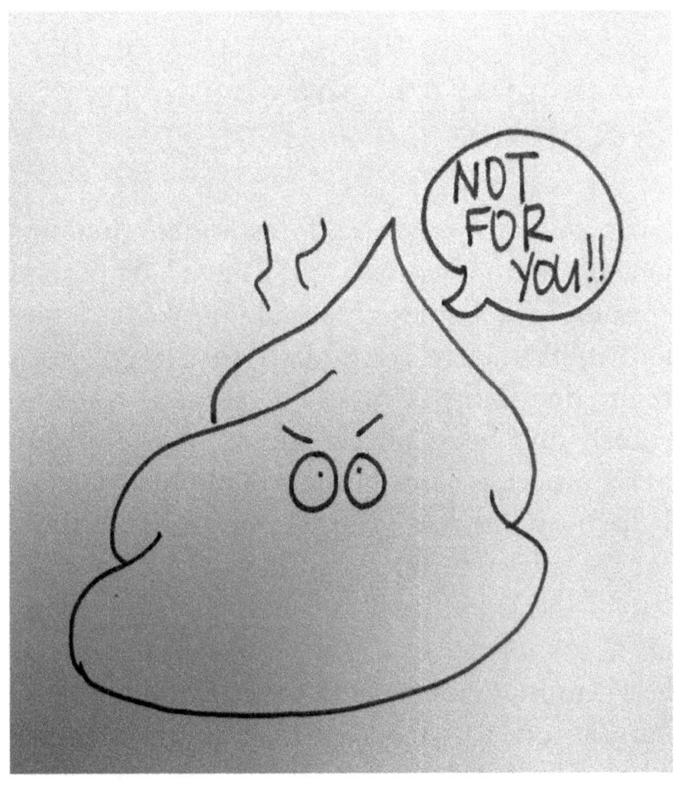

9

AM I A BAD PERSON IF I DON'T THINK ALL BABIES ARE CUTE?

According to sexist, old fashioned thinking, because I am a woman and I have lady parts, I should love babies. I should look at babies and think they're adorable, I should coo over their tiny baby clothes, I should want to squish and love all of them. Am I a bad person because I don't? Don't get me wrong, I love my nieces and nephews, and think they're adorable (because they are). I love my friends' kids, and will be slightly jealous if my alien spawn doesn't come out as cute as the last one my friend made. But I don't find all babies cute. In fact, a lot of them look like Benjamin Button, which freaks me out a little. As for baby clothes, they don't send me into vapors. Sure, I get excited when I find a Cheshire Cat onesie, or one that has 80's slasher movie chibis on it, but let's be honest – I would have rather found one that's my size. If I could dress my kid in Horror and Sci-Fi tee shirts every day, that's good enough for me. Actually, that makes me wonder…can I turn spare t-shirts into baby clothes? I'll have to remember to check on that.

But for all you out there, please don't expect me to coo over or want to carry your baby, just because I have one baking. I don't. I'll love my alien, and my friends' offspring, because they're family. But I'm not going to fake baby fever for you. Instead, let's talk about the newest J.K. Rowling Harry Potter bombshell, or debate whether Rey is related to Luke Skywalker, or play some games. I'm still a person, with my same interests and dislikes (and some hormone feelings thrown into the mix). I promise not to ask you how adorable you think my kid is. And if I do, please be honest. Because looks aren't everything. Most babies look like weird little old men….even mine probably will. Or they look like aliens. And they have gross crusty scalps. No one tells you about the crusty scalp before you have the kid, because it'll gross you out. Freshly baked babies aren't cute. In fact, they're mostly like little Play doh blob babies. That's why you have to stick the bow on your kid, because even though we pretend, we really don't know if it's a girl or a boy.   It looks like a little bald wrinkly thing. The older they get, the cuter they get. If you want an honest opinion from me, ask me about your kid when it's over a year old, looks like a tiny human, and has a personality of sorts.

Post Baby disclaimer: Geeky baby clothes are fun, and I've spent way more than I care to admit on Star Wars onesies. But why does all girl stuff have to be pink? Ugh. I still don't want to hold your kid thought. And while I may show you pictures of my offspring (who thankfully doesn't look like an alien, although she was kind of Benjamin Button-y), I would still rather talk about my podcast, or whether J.K. Rowling's post-Potter books hold a candle to the adventures of Harry and Co., or play some games….although thanks to tiny Miss Grabby Hands, I don't get to do a lot of that.

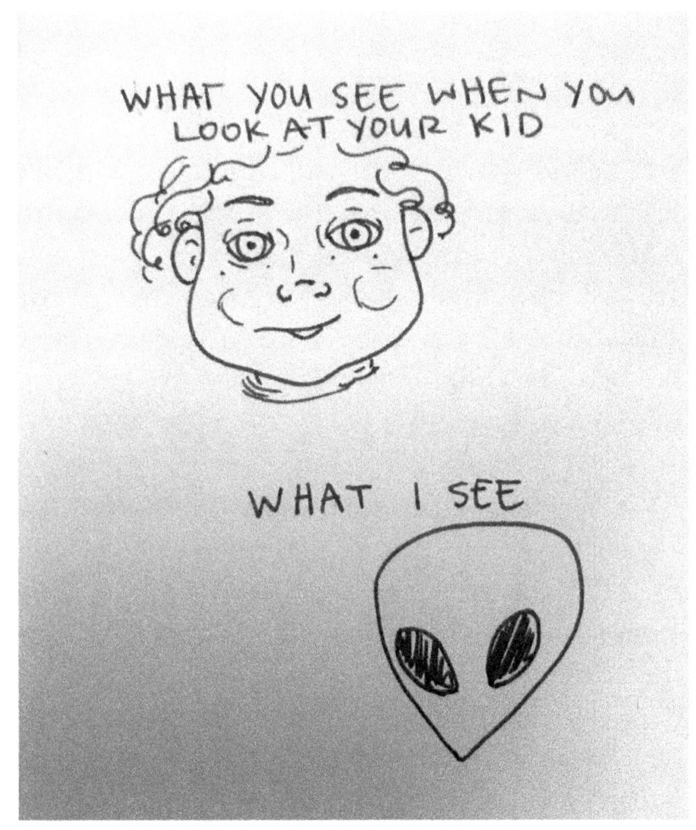
WHAT YOU SEE WHEN YOU
LOOK AT YOUR KID
WHAT I SEE

10
ADULT DIAPERS:
NOT JUST FOR THE COOL KIDS

Do you work somewhere where, whenever you need to answer the call of nature, you can just stand up, walk to the nearest restroom, and relieve yourself? If you answered yes, you are a lucky, lucky person. (Also, thanks for answering! I hate when I ask a question and no one answers….it's one of the worst parts of teacher lecture life.)

As a teacher, I get to pee in the 10 minute breaks between classes…if there isn't a line for the nearest teacher bathroom. It's a statistical fact that whenever you need to go the worst, everyone else in the hall will also be in desperate need of the facilities, so it becomes a race for the ONE teacher bathroom in our hall of 12-14 adults. Factor in the time it takes for your room to clear, plus travel time, I get about 45 seconds to actually use the restroom before I have to race back and open my classroom before the bell rings. I've always been a big coffee drinker – plus I try to drink at least 48 ounces of water during work every day – so I made that trek every time the bell rang, hoping against hope that there wasn't a line of teachers waiting before me.

That was then.

Now, thanks to my tiny alien pressing on my bladder, I need to pee every five minutes. Have a sip of water? Need to pee. Cup of tea? Need to pee. The hour and a half long periods I'm trapped in the classroom during have become torturous. I do the pee pee dance, hop from foot to foot, pace while doing kegels….anything I can do to keep from wetting myself in front of the kids. Every week the baby grows, the need to go gets worse. All the literature encourages you DRINK LOTS OF WATER! but they don't take into account the sincere need I have to not pee my pants in front of a bunch of high school students. As I browsed the irregularity aisle my eye chanced upon the display of adult diapers, shining like a beacon….and I was really tempted to buy a package and rock those puppies with pride. I would be Lexie Grey and Cristina Yang from Grey's Anatomy (remember, I was binge watching all the shows) and rock my granny diapers. Others would gasp with amazement and exclaim

"Look at her, the amazing camel woman! She can drink a 24 ounce bottle of water without having to dash to the potty! See her have 2 drinks in a period – with NO effect!" Yep, those diapers would change my life. Of course, I'll probably never end up buying them, for multiple reasons. One, it would be really hard to hide the fact that I'm wearing diapers in my yoga pants - remember my yoga pants? We covered that already. And two, because I live in fear of smelling…and when I rocked a fancy adult diaper, how can I be sure I don't smell like a urinal? But still, it's a nice dream.

I'm a teacher, and we had a lock down the other day. For those of you who don't have regular active shooter drills, a lockdown is just what it sounds like – you are locked in your room/office because there is an immediate threat, and you have to remain there until it's been cleared. In a drill, this takes about 15 minutes. This time, we were locked down for 2 hours…..during which I had the tiny parasite acting out the mambo scene from Dirty Dancing on my bladder. There was nothing I could do. We have an "emergency bucket" but there's no way that thing was getting broken in. I spent half the time cursing my decision to not rock adult diapers. I mean, why not? I wear skirts. Who would know? Tomorrow, I just might.

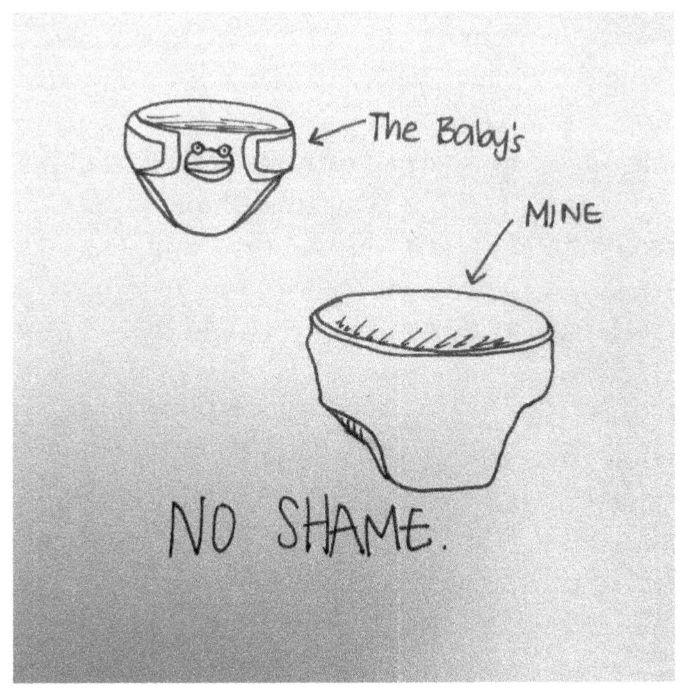

11
LET'S BRING BACK NAPS

I'm tired - all the time, I could fall asleep right here writing this right now tired. I'm blaming a lot of my exhaustion on the fact that I'm growing a human. Since before I even knew I was pregnant, this tiny little alien inside me has caused my energy levels to plummet. I take naps right after I get home from work. I struggle to stay awake after 1 pm on any day. I get tired going to the market, or walking across campus, or breathing. It's ridiculous. At work, I get a half hour lunch, but I'm never able to rest during that time because there are always people in my room. On weekends, I'll go to the store, and by the time I get home I'm so tired I could use a good lie down. The fact that I can't have my typical cups of coffee doesn't help with my eternal fatigue. My bag of Death Wish Coffee stares at me from my freezer, calling to me when I'm at my most tired.

This is all exacerbated by the fact that I can't sleep through the night. Between the eternal numbness in my hands and the alien twinges in my belly, deep sleep has eluded me. I toss and turn, reach for the iPad in the hope that

Netflix will lull me back to sleep, and then eventually give up and wander over to the sofa to stare into space. It's an ongoing struggle, and so far insomnia is winning.

I would like to crack jokes about my extreme exhaustion and lack of sleep turning me into a zombie, but I'm too freaking tired.

I wish we could adopt the afternoon siesta, like they do in other countries. Let's take a two hour break in the middle of the day, for lunch and naps. Five minutes to eat a yogurt, and then an hour and a half for sweet, sweet sleep. It would make the work day so much better. That pesky post-lunch exhaustion would be a thing of the past – no more attempting to make words and fake energy while heartily wishing my desk was a bed. On that note, why don't they make desks that pull out into beds? They make sofa beds. Someone should totally make a desk bed - I'd buy that sucker in a heartbeat.

People keep telling me to rest now, because when the baby comes I won't get any sleep. Have these people never been pregnant? Let say that I was used to sleeping on my back, which I'm not - 100% stomach sleeper over here. So assuming I could easily fall asleep, my tiny unborn human has decided that two to three AM is the optimal time to have a dance party. I think her dance style of choice is somewhere between "mosh pit" and "breakdancing". All I know is it involves a lot of beating up my other organs. How am I supposed to sleep through that? I guess I'll just have to wait and sleep when I'm dead...or when the tiny one goes off to college.

Until then, I'll be over here, trying not to fall asleep as you're talking.

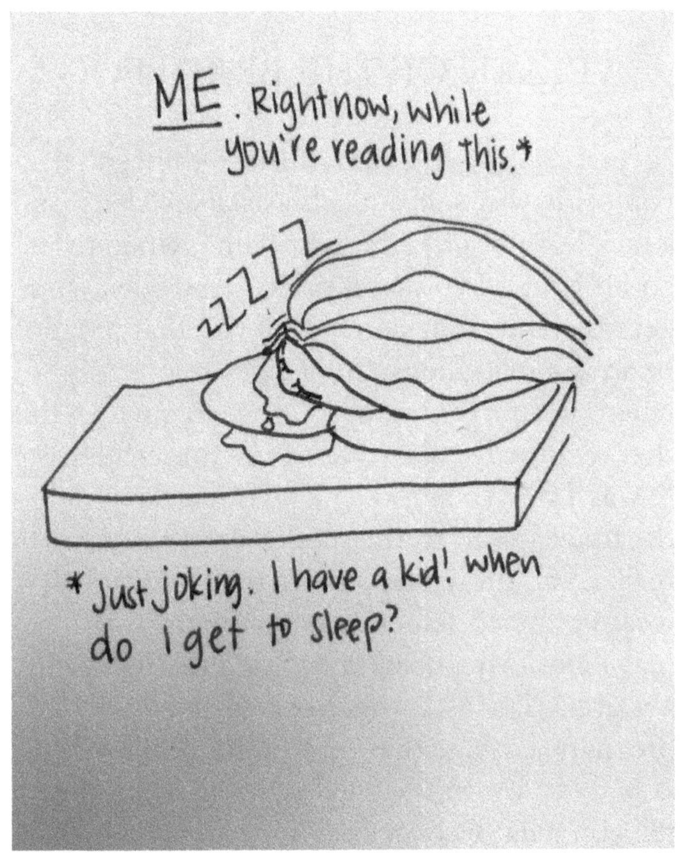

ME. Right now, while you're reading this.*
zZZZZ
* Just joking. I have a kid! when do I get to sleep?

12
ATTACK OF THE BRAIN FOG

Mental Acuity. It's one of those things that you pride yourself on. Phrases like "sharp as a tack" or "bright as a light bulb", when used about you, fill you with pride. And then, you get pregnant. I'm here to tell you that preggo brain is a real thing. Pre-alien, I might forget where I put my keys every once in a while, but that was the usual extent of my forgetfulness. Now, I'm a total mess. The other day, I left the house to go to the market…and then realized about halfway there that I was wearing my cookie monster slippers instead of real shoes. My husband mocked me for days about it. This is another one of those pregnancy things that they either don't tell you about or drastically downplay when they tell you what to expect.

My brain fog was bad. One day I put my pants on backwards, and then spent hours wondering why, all of a sudden, they didn't cover my bum anymore (and these weren't my fat pants – these were my super pricy Lula Roe leggings that fit you even though if you eat an entire Thanksgiving meal). I've forgotten where I put my keys more times than I can count, and I've lost 2 credit cards.

I still have no idea where they are. They're probably next to my other car key, on my really mice lanyard.

I think my poor husband is starting to think I'm mental. I'll tell him something, only to get "yeah, you told me" in response….but I don't remember telling him at all. Or I'll think I told him something, assume I did, and then get grumpy that he doesn't know what I'm talking about. I ask the same questions multiple times. And, the worst, considering my job, I'll be talking about something and then just trail off. It's not too bad if I'm talking to the man or one of my friends that is used to my brain fog, but it's super unhelpful when I'm trying to lecture on World War 1. "The Battle of Tannenburg was a significant event because………". It's cool, children, you can fill in the blanks, right? I forget simple words like "war" or "handout" – words that I use every day at work. My once smooth instruction giving takes way longer now, and I have to struggle at times to think of what I should be doing.

I'm hoping that once the baby is done baking, the brain fog that has attacked my poor cranium will dissipate and I'll be back to my old self, because I really can't afford to lose any more credit cards. And until the fashion world decides that slippers are the height of fashion, I should probably avoid wearing them out in public (and walking the dog doesn't count). If it doesn't, well, I'll become of those crazy old ladies with scarves way earlier than I was planning.

Post baby update: The brain fog did finally lift a little. I haven't worn my slippers to the market since the tiny one was born. However, (and this is another thing they don't tell you) the pregnancy brain fog is replaced by post-baby-no-sleep-exhaustion.

And I still haven't found my credit cards or my keys.

Or, You Thought This Was Going To Be Easy?

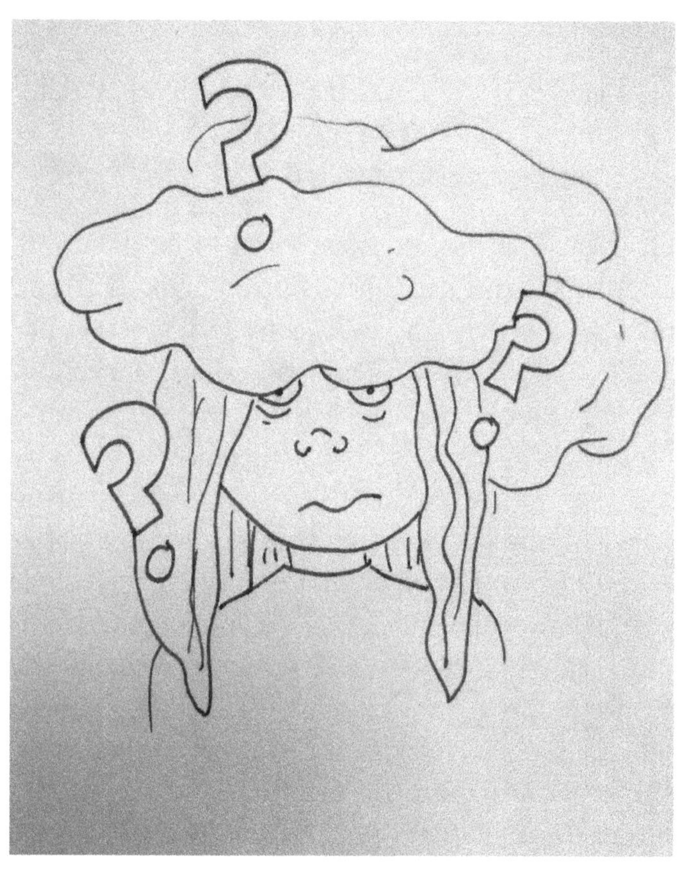

13
WHEN SEX TAKES ON A WHOLE NEW MEANING

Do you remember when you used to think about sex, and it conjured up images of naked people, sweaty fun, and an overall good time? That, of course, was pre-alien insertion. Now, whenever people talk about sex around me, it has nothing to do with naked time, and more with whether or not my future offspring has a penis. Everyone wants to know what you're having when you're expecting, and if you don't want to know, they take it as a personal affront. How dare you not know the gender of your baby? How will people know whether to get girly pink shit or rugged blue shit? Never mind the fact that you might not buy into all of that "girls have to be girly, guys have to play with trucks stuff". People want to know what color shit to buy.

As I make my way through baby registries and stores to stock up in advance of my parasite's arrival, it's hard to ignore all of the blue and pink everywhere. And if you want to avoid those, or, heaven forbid, want to be surprised, you have your choice of yellow or green.

Because those are the only colors left. It's depressing.

This, inevitably, leads to the "gender reveal" party – one of the newest and most popular things to waste money on before your baby is born - balloons in a box, or a color in a cake, or a myriad of other ways to let people know what you're having. If it's done at your baby shower, you're still depriving people of knowing what stereotype to shop for…and if it's a separate party, really? Do you need to different parties? Use that extra money to buy supplies for your kid – diapers are expensive! Of course, there are less expensive ways to inform people what kind of genitals your kid will have. You can do a cutesy picture, or post a poll and reveal results. We let people guess on Facebook, then greyed out the sex the baby wasn't.

I'm having a girl, which means that people are already talking about how my kid will want to be a princess, or a fairy, or a ballerina. Let's totally overlook that this kid will be raised by two horror loving Star Wars geeks, and my favorite color is black. Honestly, our kid will be more likely to want to be a Stormtrooper and do martial arts like her dad then grow up to be like Tinkerbell. Or think that black chucks and Doc Martins are appropriate footwear, like her mom. And who knows? She might grow up and decide she's a boy. And that's okay too. Because who are we do force our kid to be a girly girl just because she has girl parts, or a dude because he's got a penis? The kid should be able to do what he or she wants. My brothers have already bought mine a bunch of boy onesies, and that's okay. Because in the long run, what really matters is that the kid is alive and happy. Who cares what color or style clothes or toys the kid has.

Now, excuse me while I go hang up the Black Widow costume and Cheshire Cat onesie I got for my baby.

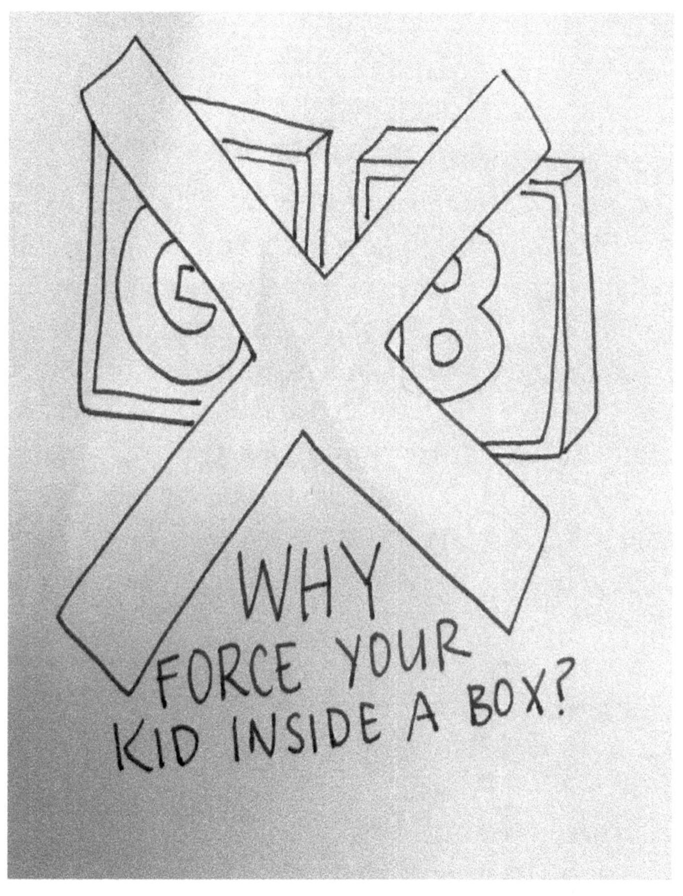
WHY
FORCE YOUR
KID INSIDE A BOX?

14
HOW COME EVERYONE HAS A BUMP BUT ME?

Let's talk about pregnancy envy. Before I got pregnant, I was okay with myself. Sure, I could definitely be a lot skinnier and more toned, and I have a slightly witchy nose. But overall, I was okay. I'll admit to some envy when I saw a lady with super perky boobs or really toned arms, but there was no raging green eyed monster living inside of me. Now that I'm pregnant, of course, that has all changed. All body envy bets are off. And it has nothing to do with my jiggly arms, or my booty, or even my saggy boobs. Nope – this is straight up tummy envy. Where I used to look at my flab and wish I had those rock hard abs like the chick on the cover of Women's health, now I wish I looked like I was actually pregnant at all.

I belong to at least one mommy-to-be message board (okay, like 4), and read all the pregnancy blogs I can. One thing all of them have, along with every woman I see in person that is pregnant, is a nice baby bump. A full, "I just swallowed this bowling/beach ball" stomach that clearly indicates "This chick is having a baby!" The other pregnant ladies at work have them, the girls at the store have them, and everyone has them – except me. I didn't look pregnant at all until I was almost 8 months….until then I had that 6 weeks pregnant " I just ate a really big meal" chubby belly. Now, with mere weeks to go, I look like I could maybe be pregnant. But it's not a good bump. It doesn't stick out, it's not round, and it doesn't scream "baby on board!!" It's just frustrating. I walk through the store, running across women who are way less pregnant but way more pregnant looking than me, and I get angry and jealous. I bet those woman don't worry that everyone around them is just assuming they're a gluttonous fatty when they eat all the food, or complain about having to walk around.

Because I'm not obviously pregnant, I worry about all of this, and more. I can't walk a lot, because it brings on contractions. I can't breathe because there's a baby squishing all my organs into uncomfortable positions. Everything hurts, and I live in constant pain. But to the casual observer, I'm just an overweight fat chick, who should maybe start exercising and cut back on her portions. And my overwhelming certainty that everyone is judging me in this manner just adds to my hardcore jealousy for all the normally pregnant ladies out there. I'm sure there are others out there who can sympathize - I'm looking at you, ladies on "I Didn't Know I was Pregnant"!

It's so frustrating to be growing a person but not be obviously growing a person. I want that glow, and that belly. I want the cute shirts with the designs on them that only make sense because they're stretched tight across your round beach ball belly. I want the belly that people have to resist rubbing because it's adorable and pregnant. Instead, I have that "I had too much salty food belly". The struggle is real.

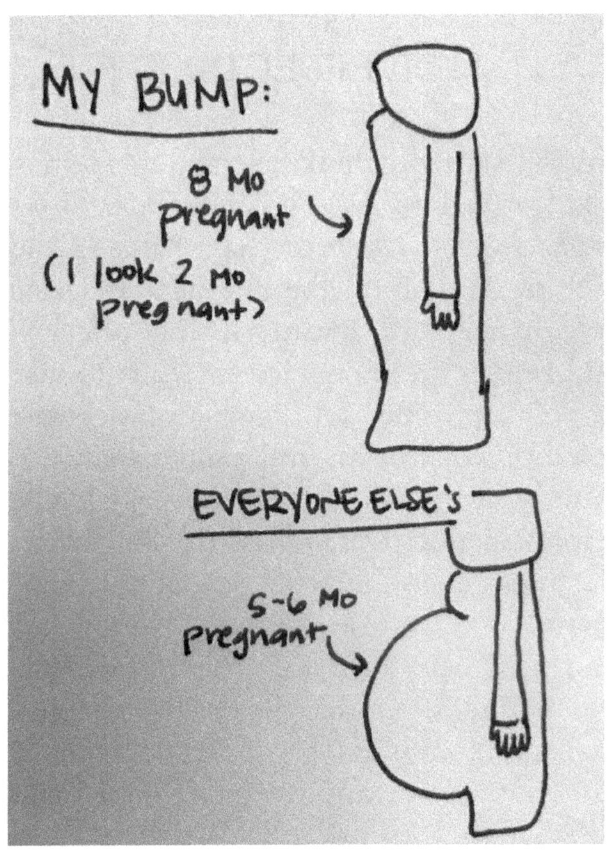
MY BUMP:
8 MO pregnant
(I look 2 mo pregnant)
EVERYONE ELSE'S
5-6 MO pregnant

15
SIDE EFFECTS

When I started thinking about getting pregnant, I read books – *What to Expect When You're Expecting, The First Time Mom* – and spent a lot of time on the internet. I started my pregnancy well aware of the effect it would have on my energy levels, ready to take on a few months of morning sickness, schooled on belly bands and pants expanders. I was ready to go. Now, with 8 weeks left to go before eviction day, I'm left thinking about all the things they don't tell you about being pregnant. I've already ranted about my inability to eat 90% of the foods out there….but at 8 months, that hasn't changed much. I can now eat about 80-85% of all foods – not a great improvement. But that's the least of the fun side effects that you can expect.

I feel like if pregnancy was a drug, it would definitely need to have one of those voiceover guys at the end. You know, the ones that rattle off all of the horrible things that can happen if you take that pill. Sure, it may cure your insomnia, but you might eat everything in your fridge or drive while fast asleep, want to kill yourself, have all of your hair fall out, or grow tentacles. (Okay, that last one probably won't happen). Pregnancy needs one of those. I've found a few sites here and there that bring these up, but mostly hidden in the "week by week" breakdown – that stuff you don't actually look at until it's too late to turn back. Pregnancy: may cause insomnia, random pains, and an inability to move freely, leg cramps, a 9 month cold, and other joyous things!

Let's talk about your nose. I'm a teacher, so I'm used to catching a bug now and then when the school becomes a breeding ground for viruses. Now, however, I feel like I've had a cold for MONTHS. And because everything you read makes you so scared to take any medicines, in case your kid comes out a flipper baby, I tried to just power through. Forget the fact that it's already hard to breathe with 45 pounds of uterus pressing on your lungs and diaphragm. Throw in a constantly stuffy nose, and the fun never stops! Plus it makes it way harder to sleep.
Ah, sleep. I look back on the days when I got 4 straight hours of sleep with nostalgia. Today, between the stuffy nose and the fact that I feel like a giant whale (albeit a whale

that gets horrible pains whenever they move), sleep is almost impossible. And if one more person tells me its "good practice for when the baby comes", I'm going to punch someone. Seriously. Because I am sleep deprived and cranky. I had read about ligament pain when I first got pregnant, but failed to grasp its seriousness. That shit hurts. I look back on my period cramps and miss that little pain, because in a day or two it was gone. Your uterus stretches forever, and each tiny growth spurt from your kid can trigger bigger and better tummy cramps. Oh, and that whale feeling? Your growing belly will make it difficult to sit, stand, roll over, or lay down. Basically, everything might hurt. I saw a woman running a half marathon a few months ago, and she was about 7 months pregnant. As I watched her run down the street, smiling, I was in awe. I couldn't run a half marathon if you paid me. And now, as I sit here further along than her, I'm in even more awe. It hurts to walk the 15 feet from my classroom to the restroom – I couldn't imagine jogging like this

I can't wait to see what last minute hidden horrors this pregnancy has in store for me.

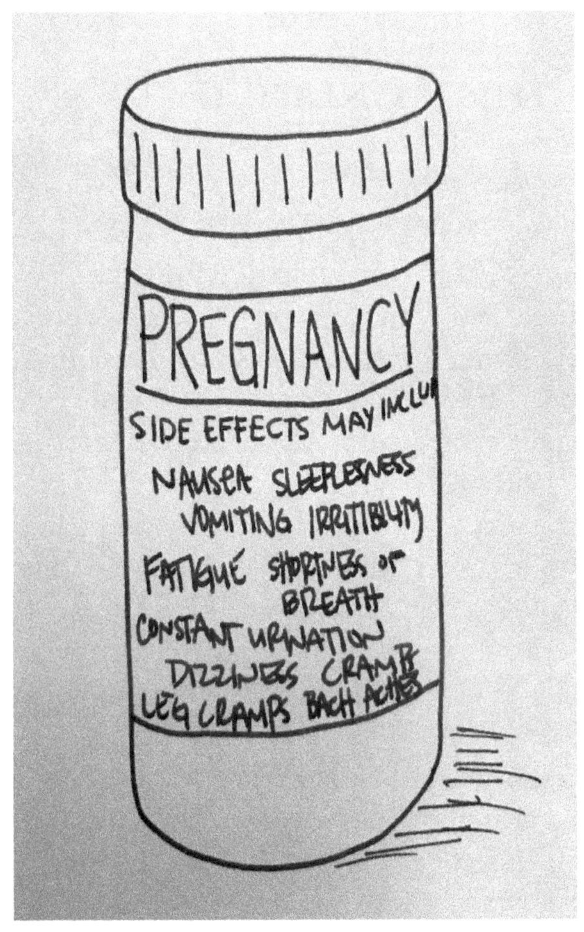

PREGNANCY
SIDE EFFECTS MAY INCLUDE
NAUSEA SLEEPLESSNESS
VOMITING IRRITIBILITY
FATIGUE SHORTNESS OF
BREATH
CONSTANT URINATION
DIZZINESS CRAMPS
LEG CRAMPS BACK ACHES

16
THIS IS ONLY A TEST

In movies, when a lady starts to get contractions, her water breaks, and she's hours away from pushing a baby out. No false labor, no Braxton hicks….you know, those charming little contractions that don't signal that the end is near – they're just, according to literature, your body's way of getting ready. I call BS on this cheerful statement. You know what an eight month pregnant woman doesn't need? 20 plus contractions a day that feel like the worst period cramps ever, and make it impossible while they're happening to talk – which, when you have to lecture in class for a living, isn't very helpful or fun at all. With six weeks left until eviction day, the thought of having to deal with this every day for the next six weeks makes me want to curl up into a ball and cry. (Of course, I can't curl up, because of my giant fat preggo body….but I digress). Does every woman have this experience? Or is this another of those major suck side effects that I'm getting to deal with that the average pregnant woman is blissfully ignorant about? Inquiring minds want to know.

I have gone to Labor and Delivery 3 times in the past 3 weeks, convinced I was going into labor, thanks to some super long, drawn out, painful contractions. Each time, the doctors and nurses patted my head and assured me that these were just "mild Braxton Hicks" contractions. None of the manuals I read prepared me for this. These suckers hurt. My doctor just put me on medical leave because I literally can't walk around anymore without wanting to cry, throw up, or fall over. And I still have 6 weeks to go. I can't even be snarky about this one, folks. I don't even want to know what real labor is going to be like, if this is "mild fake labor". That's like chopping off my arm with a rusty butter knife, then patting my head and saying, "it's okay, dearie, and it's just a little flesh wound".

Legit. When the time comes, I'm totally not going to be about that natural birth. I want all of the birthing drugs. I would like to not feel the giant parasite being pushed out of my body. I'm all for the miracle of childbirth, but the same way I'm for camping – I'll do it, but I'd really like to have an inflatable mattress under my sleeping bag, a flush toilet and shower, and one of those stoves so I can cook a proper meal. I want to enjoy roughing it. I know people talk about having quick and easy childbirth, but if my labor is anything like my pregnancy has been, it won't be pretty.

Whether you choose to get an epidural when you have a baby, rock a water birth, or anything else you want to do, you rock that shit. I'm going to focus on getting through these next 6 weeks without losing my shit.

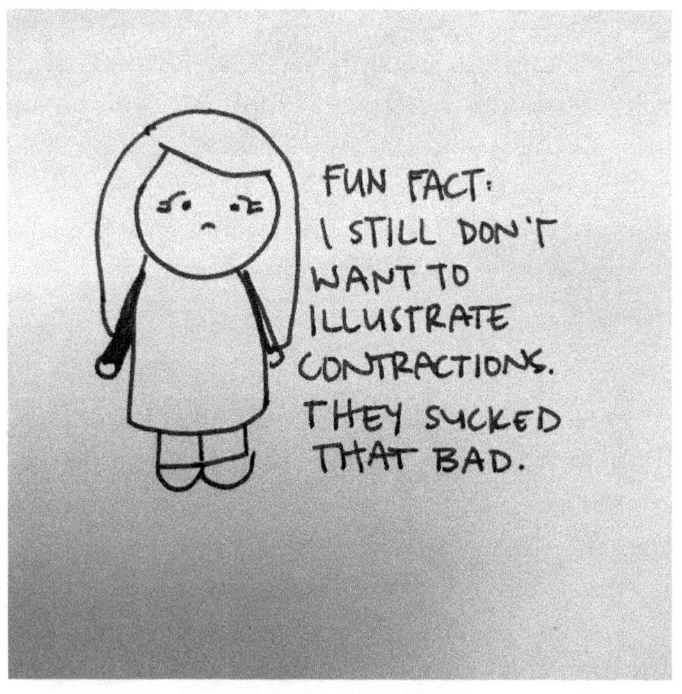

17

EVICTION NOTICE

The time has finally come.   You've survived 40 weeks (or however long you've been pregnant....some babies want to come out earlier or later).   It's time for your tiny parasite to head on out and join the world of the air breathing.

There are many ways you can rock your labor. You can labor at home, naturally. You can have a water birth. You can go to a birthing center and bounce on a yoga –excuse me – birthing ball to get the baby out. Or you can go to a hospital and do it the traditional way. Whichever way you're planning to have things go down, chances are you've been planning for a while, making arrangements, packing your bag, taking tours of the center (if you're not doing a home birth), ordering equipment (if you are). Most people get to let their baby tell them when it's ready to come out – the contractions start, the water might break, and then the little one heads for the light like they're Carol Ann in Poltergeist.

In my case, thanks to my "elderly uterus" (I'm

35) my tiny parasite couldn't linger a day past 40 weeks, so if she didn't emerge by her due date, they were going to make her emerge. That's another one of those things they don't tell you – that being a normal aged woman actually means that you have the insides of a haggard old crone. Of course, my stubborn little one refused to come out on time, so 40 weeks found me checking into the hospital to be induced, which is a fancy way of saying they were trying to torture my body in hopes that I'd magically start going into labor.

My poor put upon husband curled himself up in a chair that claimed to recline while I spent 30 hours with an epidural, itchy skin (thanks, morphine!) and Chopped on Netflix.

….and then my epidural wore off and I finally got to the point where they thought she was going to come out. 5 hours, lots of screaming, more Chopped, and - nothing. The sucker didn't want to move. I found myself whisked into an operating room for an emergency C-section, and faster than anything there was a crying gooey tiny person.

All of the books and websites tell you to pack a huge bag and make a plan. But you never know what's going to happen, so while a plan is great, being able to go with the flow is better. And I packed a bag full of all those things that the blogs told me were essential for my hospital stay, but thanks to the way my visit to Labor and Deliver went, I didn't even get to bring it.

So here's my recommendation of what you're going to need:

- Your own pillow. Hospital pillows suck.
- An iPad – hospital TV sucks. And it'll double as the music player if you made one of those "labor playlists"
- Chapstick
- A maxi skirt for when you leave the hospital – if you gave birth naturally it'll hide the diaper, and if you had a C-section it won't hurt your incision.
- Snacks – because you never know how long you're going to be there (or if the hospital food is going to suck….are you sensing a theme?)

Whatever happens, just go with it, and don't forget to breathe. Godspeed.

EVICTION·NOTICE

Dear Baby,
Your 40 weeks are up.
It's time to GTFO of my
uterus and into a crib.
Sincerely,
Management

18

CONGRATULATIONS!

YOU SURVIVED!

You successfully got that tiny parasite out of your body. Now comes the fun part – figuring how to feed him (do you breastfeed? Bottle feed? Pump then bottle? How do you know if the freaking kid is getting enough to eat??), put onesies on that tiny fragile body, and try to keep it alive. I can't tell you how many times in that first week I worried that I was going to break an arm or squish her head getting her clothes on, and don't get me started on the struggle that was breastfeeding – but that's a whole different story.

But for now, pat yourself on the back. You made it 9 months carrying a really cute parasite, and (hopefully) it didn't emerge like the chestburster in Alien. Have a drink, take a nap…..because now the fun really starts.

71

ABOUT THE AUTHOR

Sarah is a caffeine addict, crazy doodler, and mom to a tiny force of nature. She thought teaching was challenging until she tried pregnancy – which was way harder.
Sarah is the owner of SpookyDoodles Shop on Etsy, is a member of the 501st legion, reads all the books, and has zero free time. One day she'll actually get to take a nap.
She lives in Los Angeles with her husband and daughter.
She is also one of the hosts of the podcast FanFickingTastic.